Blood Pressure Tracker

Keep Your Notes In One Place

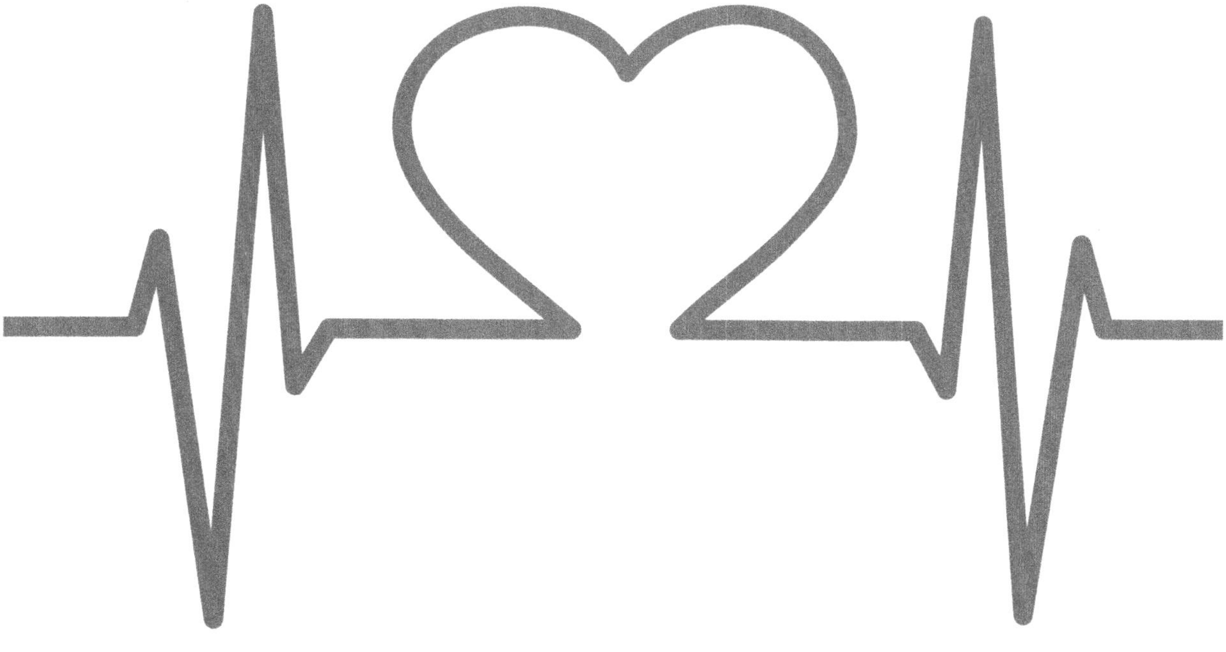

Life Log Books

First Printing

This book does not replace medical advice, nor is it intended for anything medical beside tracking.

ISBN: 978-0692728918

Dedication

This book is dedicated to the folks who spend time monitoring their blood pressure. I hope this helps you.

Important Information

My Name ______________________________

My Phone Number ______________________

My Address ___________________________

____

Allergies ____________________________

____

Additional Important Information

____

____

My Doctor's Name and Phone Number

____

____

Blood Pressure Log

date	time	systolic	diastolic	pulse
	Sample Page			
1/1/15	8am	119	79	606pm
1/1/15	6pm	110	70	606pm
1/2/15	8am	115	75	606pm
1/2/15	6pm	118	77	606pm
1/3/15	8am	117	76	626pm
1/3/15	6pm	120	80	656pm

Weekly Check-In

How Did I Feel This Week? ______________________________

____

____

____

I Had A Reaction To...__________________________________

____

____

____

I Need To Tell My Doctor About... ____________________

____

____

____

____

I Would Like To Change... ____________________________

____

____

____

____

____

Blood Pressure Log

date	time	systolic	diastolic	pulse

Weekly Check-In

How Did I Feel This Week? ______________________

I Had A Reaction To...______________________

I Need To Tell My Doctor About... ______________________

I Would Like To Change... ______________________

Blood Pressure Log

date	time	systolic	diastolic	pulse

Weekly Check-In

How Did I Feel This Week? ____________________

I Had A Reaction To... ____________________

I Need To Tell My Doctor About... ____________________

I Would Like To Change... ____________________

Blood Pressure Log

date	time	systolic	diastolic	pulse

Weekly Check-In

How Did I Feel This Week? ______________________________

____

____

____

I Had A Reaction To...__________________________________

____

____

____

I Need To Tell My Doctor About... ________________________

____

____

____

____

I Would Like To Change... ______________________________

____

____

____

____

____

Blood Pressure Log

date	time	systolic	diastolic	pulse

Weekly Check-In

How Did I Feel This Week? ________________________________

I Had A Reaction To...________________________________

I Need To Tell My Doctor About... ________________________________

I Would Like To Change... ________________________________

Blood Pressure Log

date	time	systolic	diastolic	pulse

Weekly Check-In

How Did I Feel This Week? ________________________

I Had A Reaction To...________________________

I Need To Tell My Doctor About... ________________________

I Would Like To Change... ________________________

Blood Pressure Log

date	time	systolic	diastolic	pulse

Weekly Check-In

How Did I Feel This Week? ______________________________

____

____

____

I Had A Reaction To...__________________________________

____

____

____

I Need To Tell My Doctor About... __________________

____

____

____

____

I Would Like To Change... ________________________

____

____

____

____

____

Blood Pressure Log

date	time	systolic	diastolic	pulse

Weekly Check-In

How Did I Feel This Week? ________________

I Had A Reaction To...________________

I Need To Tell My Doctor About... ________________

I Would Like To Change... ________________

Blood Pressure Log

date	time	systolic	diastolic	pulse

Weekly Check-In

How Did I Feel This Week? ______________________

I Had A Reaction To...______________________

I Need To Tell My Doctor About... ______________________

I Would Like To Change... ______________________

Blood Pressure Log

date	time	systolic	diastolic	pulse

Weekly Check-In

How Did I Feel This Week? ______________________

I Had A Reaction To... ______________________

I Need To Tell My Doctor About... ______________________

I Would Like To Change... ______________________

Blood Pressure Log

date	time	systolic	diastolic	pulse

Weekly Check-In

How Did I Feel This Week? ____________________

I Had A Reaction To... ____________________

I Need To Tell My Doctor About... ____________________

I Would Like To Change... ____________________

Blood Pressure Log

date	time	systolic	diastolic	pulse

Weekly Check-In

How Did I Feel This Week? ______________________

____

____

____

I Had A Reaction To...___________________________

____

____

____

I Need To Tell My Doctor About... _______________

____

____

____

____

I Would Like To Change... _______________________

____

____

____

____

____

Blood Pressure Log

date	time	systolic	diastolic	pulse

Weekly Check-In

How Did I Feel This Week? ______________________________

I Had A Reaction To...______________________________

I Need To Tell My Doctor About... ______________________________

I Would Like To Change... ______________________________

Blood Pressure Log

date	time	systolic	diastolic	pulse

Weekly Check-In

How Did I Feel This Week? ______________________

____

____

____

I Had A Reaction To...__________________________

____

____

____

I Need To Tell My Doctor About... _______________

____

____

____

____

I Would Like To Change... _______________________

____

____

____

____

____

Blood Pressure Log

date	time	systolic	diastolic	pulse

Weekly Check-In

How Did I Feel This Week? ______________________________

I Had A Reaction To...______________________________

I Need To Tell My Doctor About... ______________________________

I Would Like To Change... ______________________________

Blood Pressure Log

date	time	systolic	diastolic	pulse

Weekly Check-In

How Did I Feel This Week? ______________________

____

____

____

I Had A Reaction To...__________________________

____

____

____

I Need To Tell My Doctor About... ______________

____

____

____

____

I Would Like To Change... _______________________

____

____

____

____

____

Blood Pressure Log

date	time	systolic	diastolic	pulse

Weekly Check-In

How Did I Feel This Week? ______________________

I Had A Reaction To...______________________

I Need To Tell My Doctor About... ______________________

I Would Like To Change... ______________________

Blood Pressure Log

date	time	systolic	diastolic	pulse

Weekly Check-In

How Did I Feel This Week? ______________________

I Had A Reaction To...______________________

I Need To Tell My Doctor About... ______________________

I Would Like To Change... ______________________

Blood Pressure Log

date	time	systolic	diastolic	pulse

Weekly Check-In

How Did I Feel This Week? ______________________________

I Had A Reaction To... ______________________________

I Need To Tell My Doctor About... ______________________________

I Would Like To Change... ______________________________

Blood Pressure Log

date	time	systolic	diastolic	pulse

Weekly Check-In

How Did I Feel This Week? ______________________

I Had A Reaction To...______________________

I Need To Tell My Doctor About... ______________________

I Would Like To Change... ______________________

Blood Pressure Log

date	time	systolic	diastolic	pulse

Weekly Check-In

How Did I Feel This Week?

I Had A Reaction To...

I Need To Tell My Doctor About...

I Would Like To Change...

Blood Pressure Log

date	time	systolic	diastolic	pulse

Weekly Check-In

How Did I Feel This Week? ____________________

I Had A Reaction To...____________________

I Need To Tell My Doctor About... ____________________

I Would Like To Change... ____________________

Blood Pressure Log

date	time	systolic	diastolic	pulse

Weekly Check-In

How Did I Feel This Week? ______________________

____

____

____

I Had A Reaction To...___________________________

____

____

____

I Need To Tell My Doctor About... _______________

____

____

____

____

I Would Like To Change... _______________________

____

____

____

____

____

Blood Pressure Log

date	time	systolic	diastolic	pulse

Weekly Check-In

How Did I Feel This Week? ____________________

____

____

____

I Had A Reaction To...____________________

____

____

____

I Need To Tell My Doctor About... ____________________

____

____

____

____

I Would Like To Change... ____________________

____

____

____

____

____

Blood Pressure Log

date	time	systolic	diastolic	pulse

Weekly Check-In

How Did I Feel This Week? ______________________________

I Had A Reaction To...______________________________

I Need To Tell My Doctor About... ______________________________

I Would Like To Change... ______________________________

Blood Pressure Log

date	time	systolic	diastolic	pulse

Weekly Check-In

How Did I Feel This Week? ____________________

____

____

____

I Had A Reaction To...____________________

____

____

____

I Need To Tell My Doctor About... ____________________

____

____

____

____

I Would Like To Change... ____________________

____

____

____

____

____

Blood Pressure Log

date	time	systolic	diastolic	pulse

Weekly Check-In

How Did I Feel This Week?

I Had A Reaction To...

I Need To Tell My Doctor About...

I Would Like To Change...

Blood Pressure Log

date	time	systolic	diastolic	pulse

Weekly Check-In

How Did I Feel This Week? ______________________

____

____

____

I Had A Reaction To...______________________

____

____

____

I Need To Tell My Doctor About... ______________________

____

____

____

____

I Would Like To Change... ______________________

____

____

____

____

____

Blood Pressure Log

date	time	systolic	diastolic	pulse

Made in the USA
Monee, IL
05 November 2026

67962922R10037